what am i afraid of

what am i afraid of
Poetry

Copyright © 2026 by Leslie Papp

Author: Leslie Papp
Photography: James K Papp
Illustrations: Ashton Papp

Published by Grand River Poetry Collective
Grand River Poetry Press
Grand Rapids, Michigan, USA
grandriverpoetrycollective.com

ISBN: 978-1-968226-06-0

Dedicated to all of the times that I
thought the world was going to break me

i fear beginnings

I fear the flutter when you look at me
And the sting when you don't

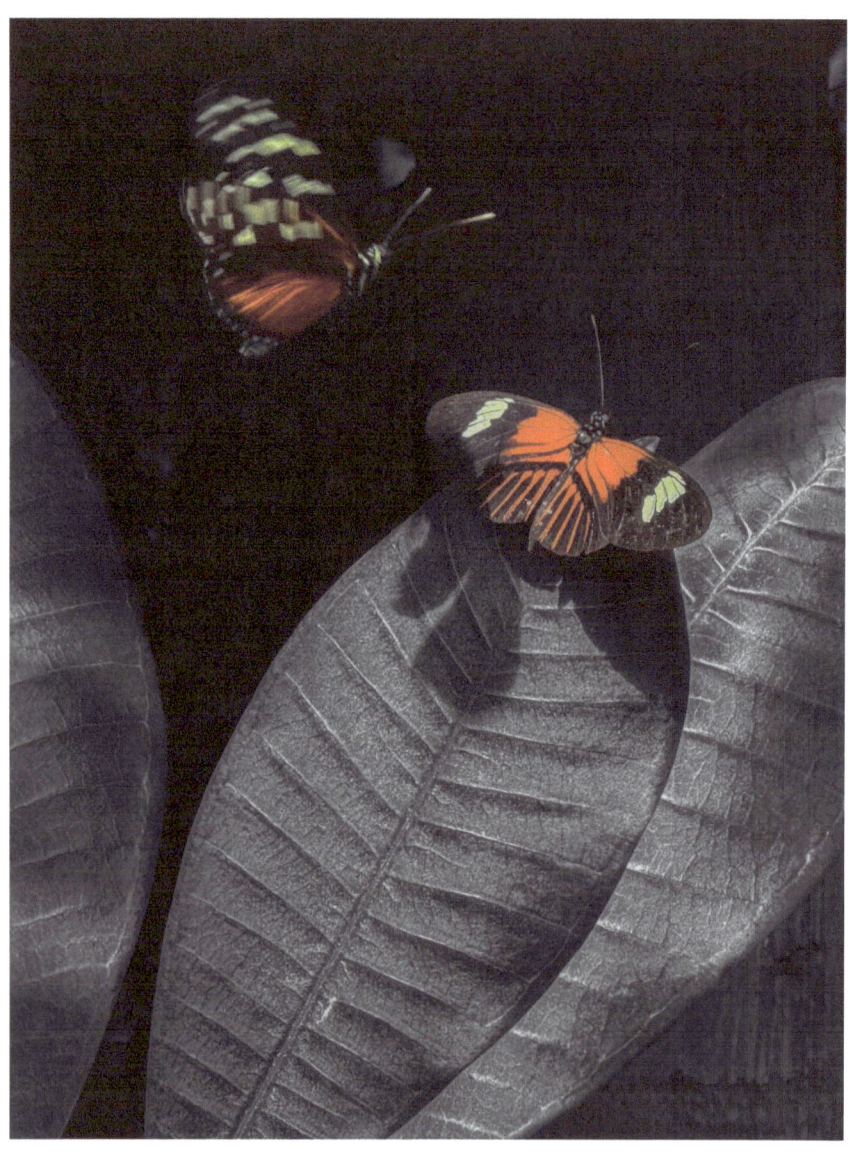

losing hold

Trying to calm my heart
As it does somersaults in my chest
Unrest birthed from violent outbursts
Winded words you breathe thin my fire
Words you say in the dark
That take on a life of their own
Each one hangs between us
By spinning threads
Moving the ground
That once held me in place

unheard

Writing is a release
A letting go of not being understood
My voice often tumbles into empty spaces
Hollow graves
Where words go to die
Buried with the souls of the unheard

what will others think

Unraveled by our doubts
A hundred breaking strands
Our tightly woven story is coming undone
Picked apart by others' eyes
To be left in a tangle of shared moments
That are no longer tethered to our hearts

giving too much

I have borders
   But no boundaries

Edges that protrude and pierce
   But do not keep me safe

I'm too much like the sun
   Stretching all parts of me
   To reach
      To touch

Everything I should not

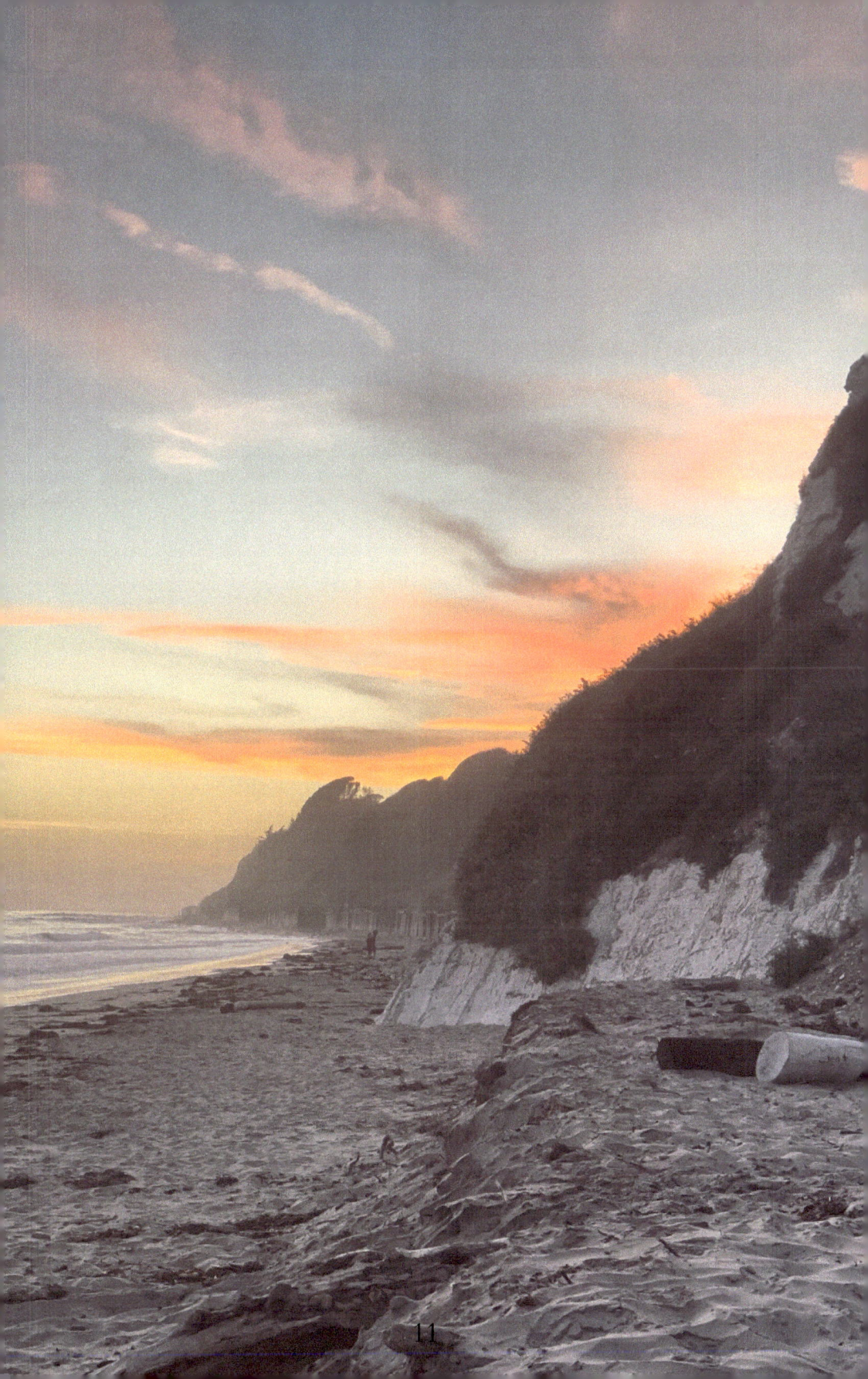

that

I'm afraid
That the love you offer me
isn't here to stay
That one day you'll decide I'm not enough
That the tides that make up my emotions
will one day take us under

I'm very afraid

I wish we could hide under the stars
Feel their heavy stillness
As the sky holds its breath

the darkness that follows the light

My days

   have turned carnivorous

Gnawing away at me

   Taking bites

   and picking fights

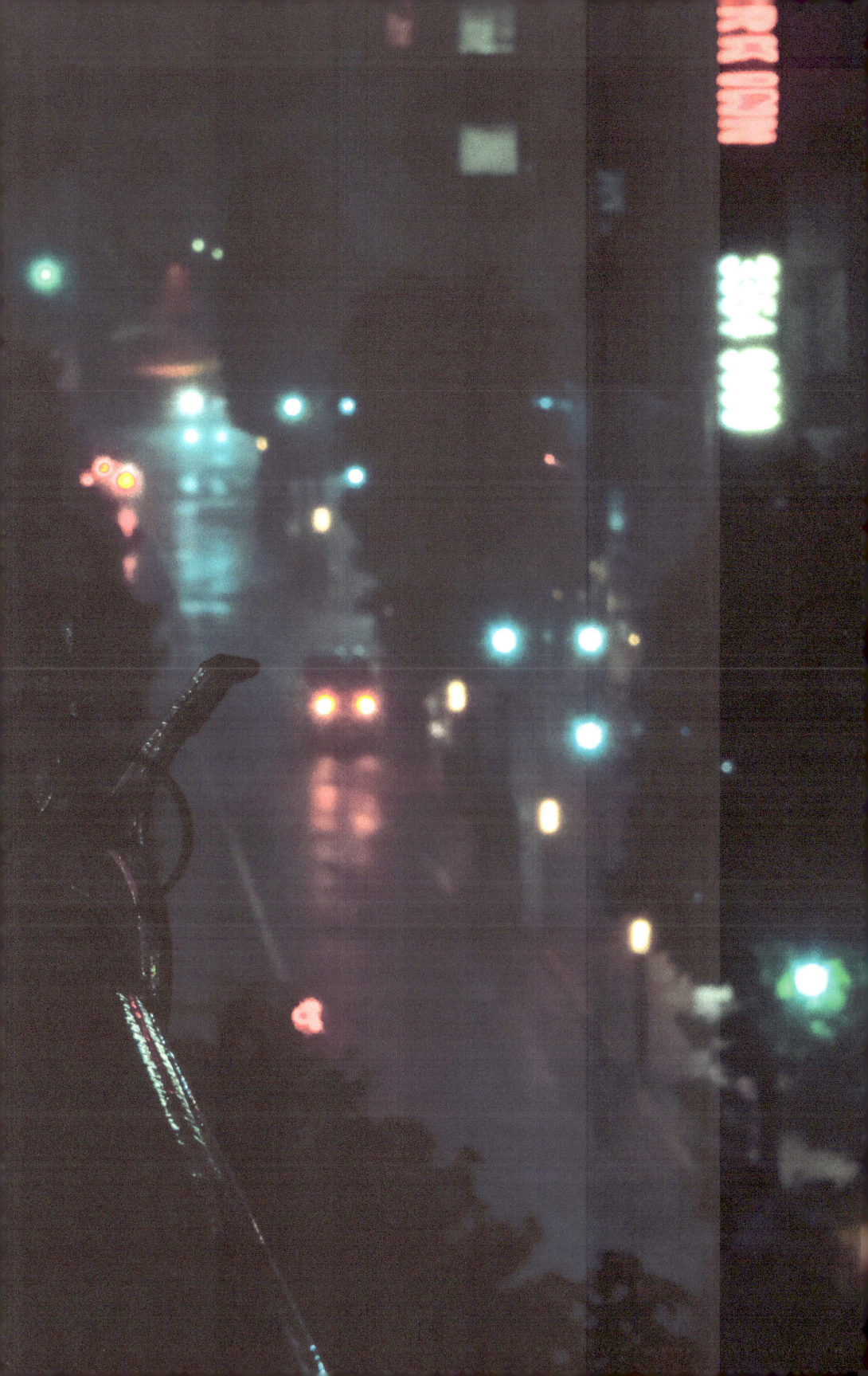

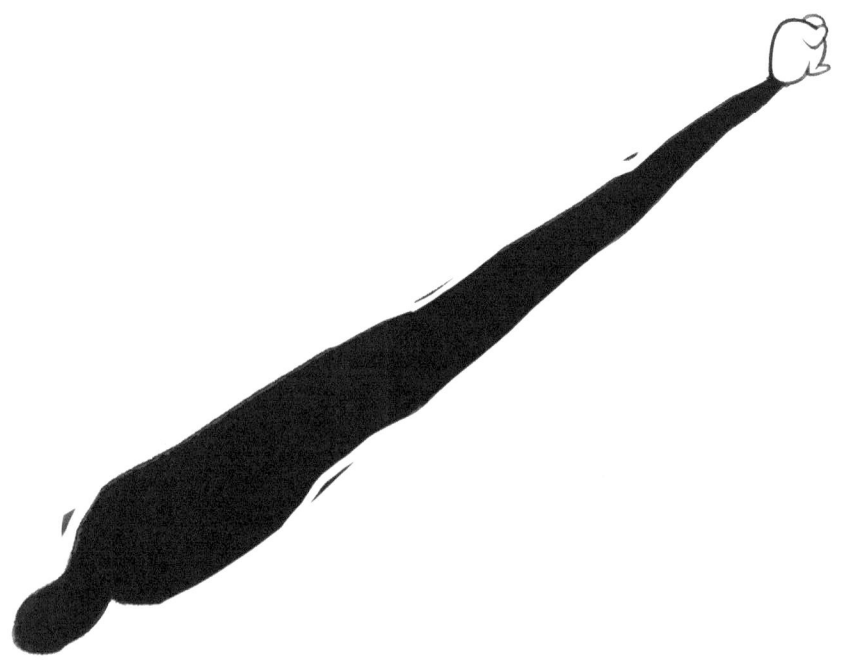

becoming the shadows

Do you ever feel like the world is too big
That you don't take up enough space
Do you ever feel like you're grabbing at walls

shrinking

To make yourself unseen

feeling like the night

As I lean over still water
Stained with the reflection of moonlit trees
My face becomes one with the sea
I become the limbs
That stand tall against the moon's smile
The mess of leaves define me,
My wants and dreams
All tangled into one night
As the wind tries to shake me free

a free fall to nowhere

Becoming too numb
All of the jabs and blows
Just become noise
As well as silence

All of the scars left behind
Grow bigger
Being fed by time

Digging deeper
To block parts of me
That were once alive

Erasing parts of me
That once let me breathe

i asked for nothing
and in return
you took everything

everything

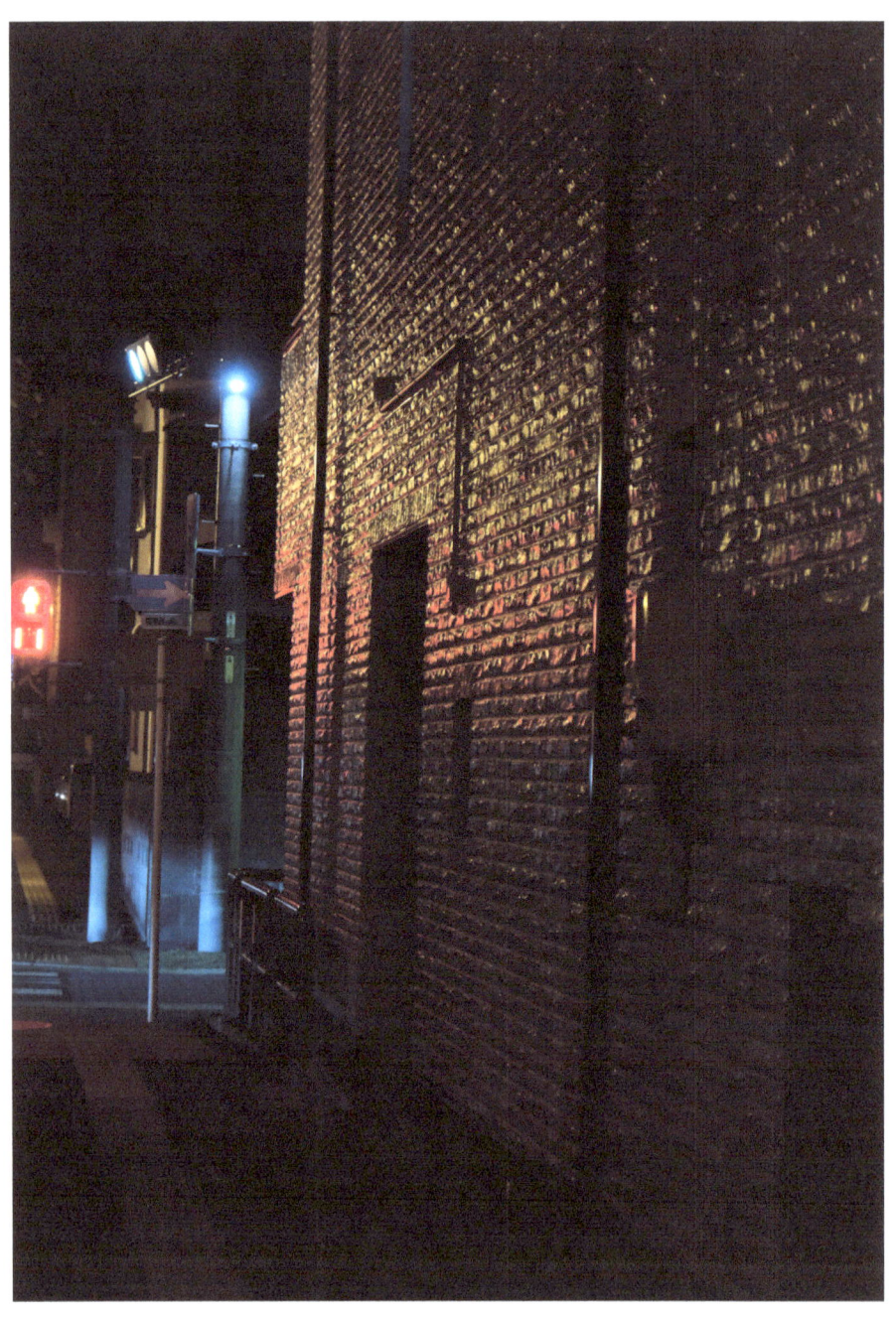

a broken heart

The drip of molten colors
Fall from hazy whiskey sunsets
And drain to the city's edge
As I slowly close my eyes on us
And am left fading to the sound
Of you walking away

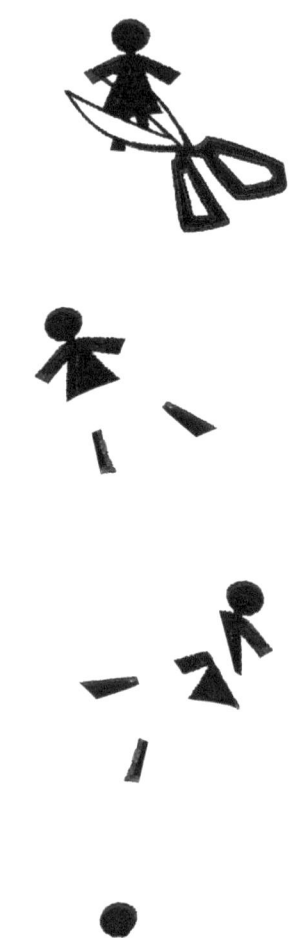

your sharp tongue

Who do you think you are
Breaking me
Into tiny
   bite-sized pieces

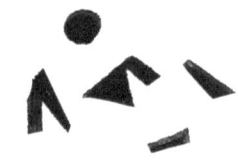

holding it all in

My body is an open space
To hold emotions
I pull out a chair for fear
And break bread with hope
Pass love around
Pretending that the dish is full
I wish to see joyfulness seated across from me
I have learned to shed tears
To clear space for happiness

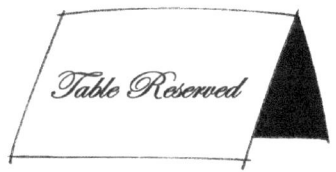

pretending

I'm bleeding from where your name has been
Carved into my heart
Etched onto my skin
Too many times of saying it under my breath
Holding my tongue
Now it seeps between my teeth
As I try to smile it all away again

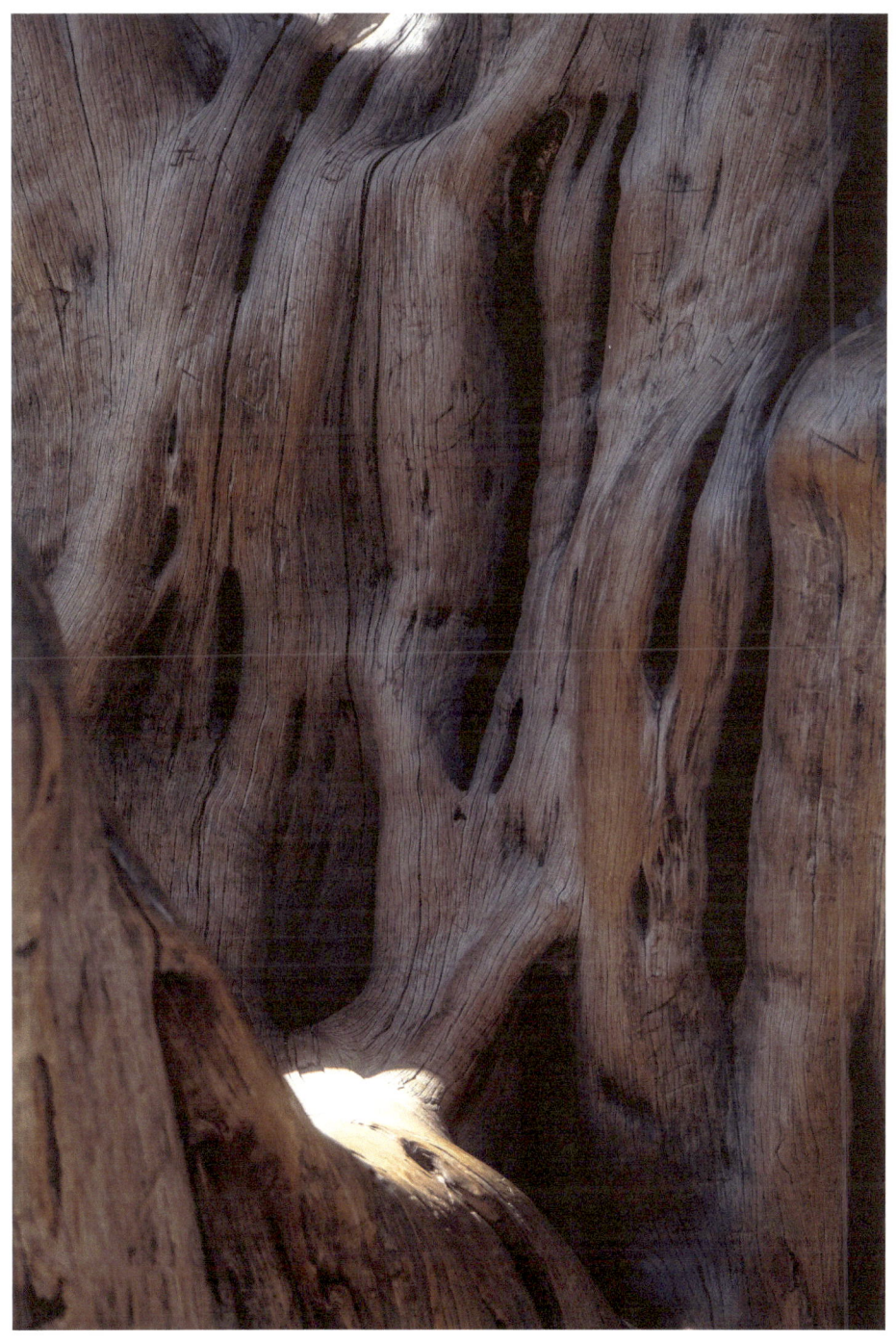

emptiness

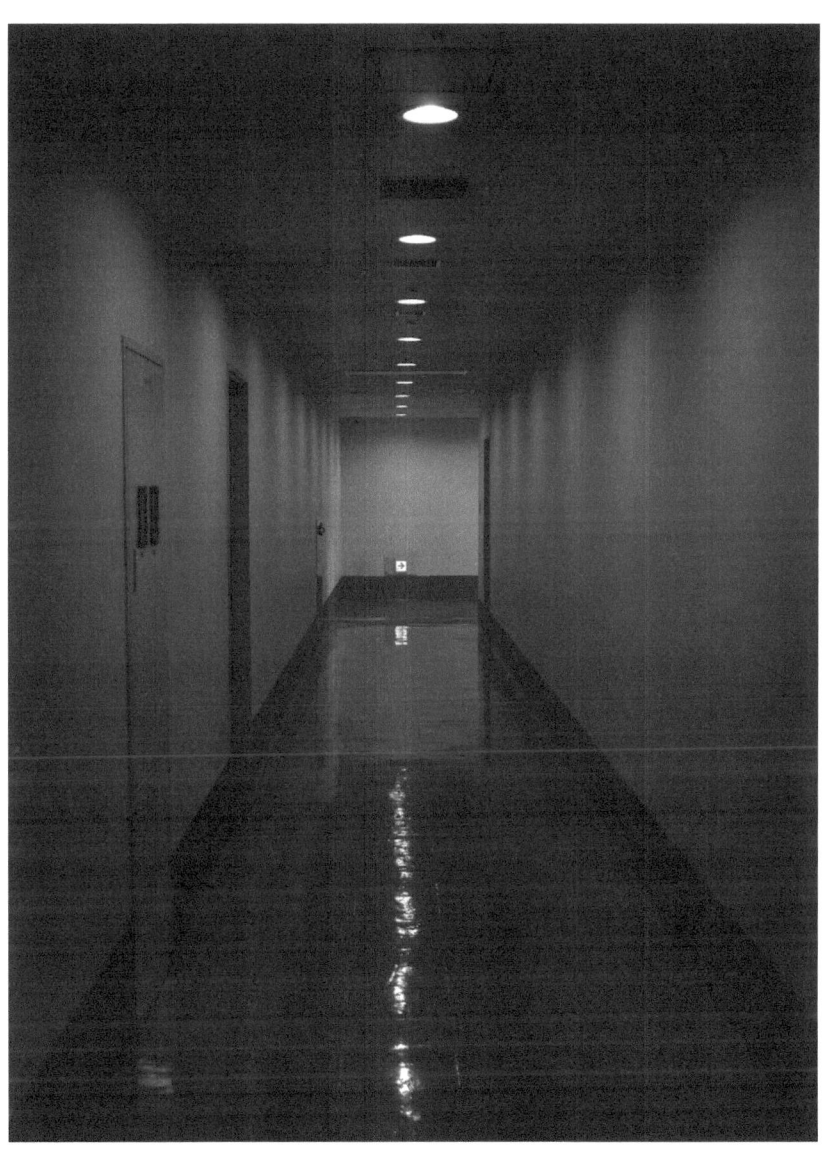

And into the darkness I went
to make peace with my ghosts

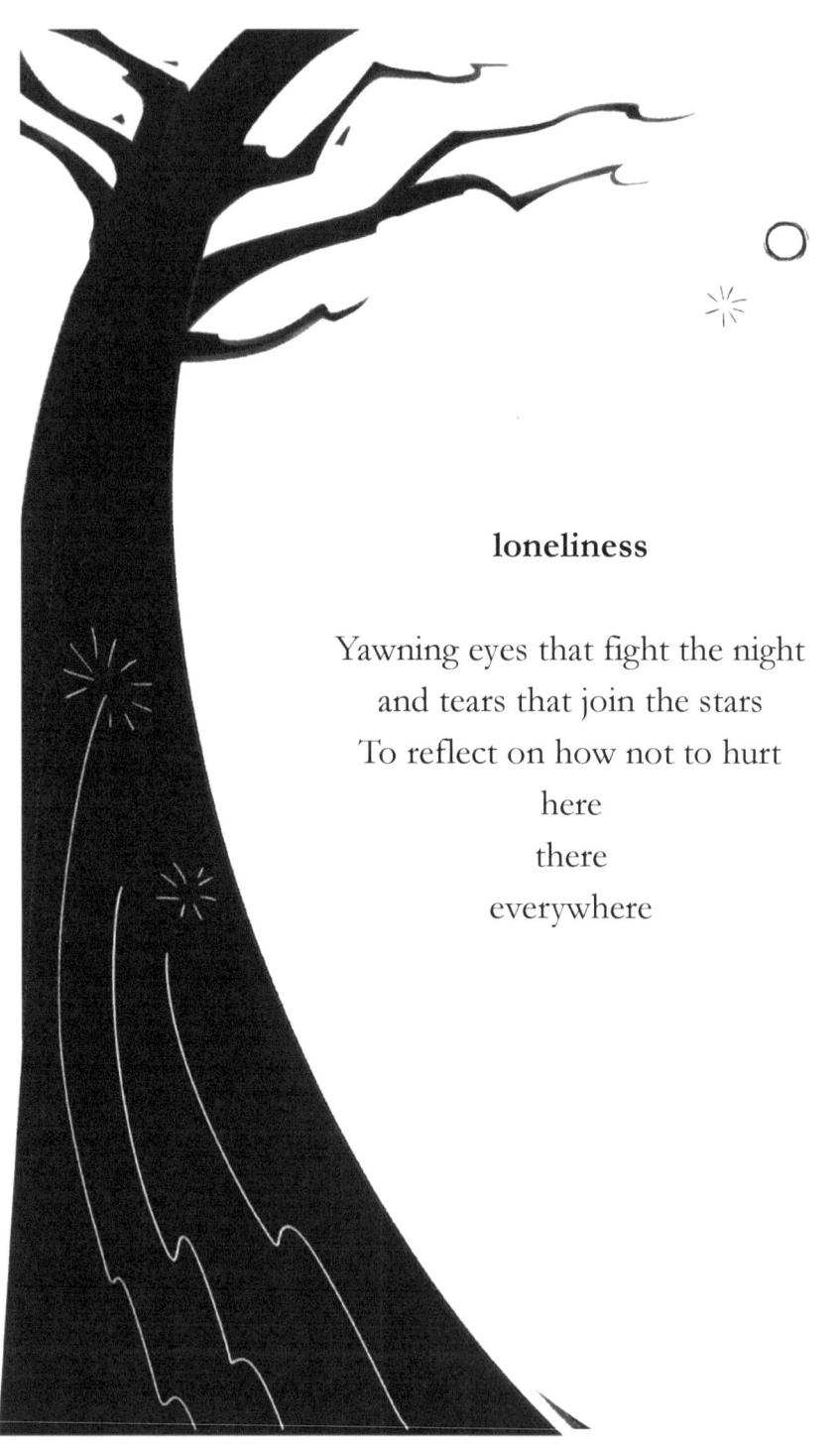

loneliness

Yawning eyes that fight the night
and tears that join the stars
To reflect on how not to hurt
here
there
everywhere

not speaking up

My mind is waning
From blaring silence
And muted still walks
I am lost within a conversation
That never happened

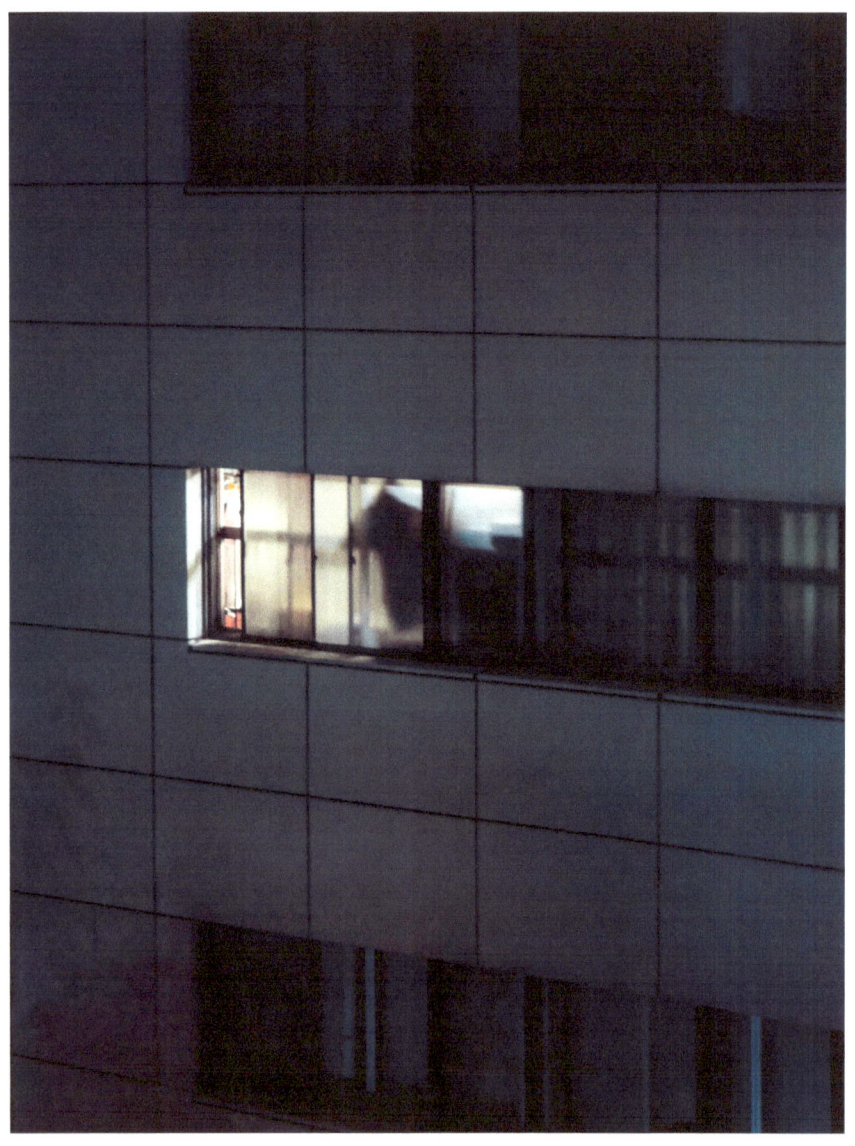

regret

I can't hurt
If I stand on the edge
Hover above the possibilities
Stay tucked away
Far from your grip
If I don't let you in
Shield myself from your touch
If I never let this become "us"
If we never begin

i'm afraid of the dark

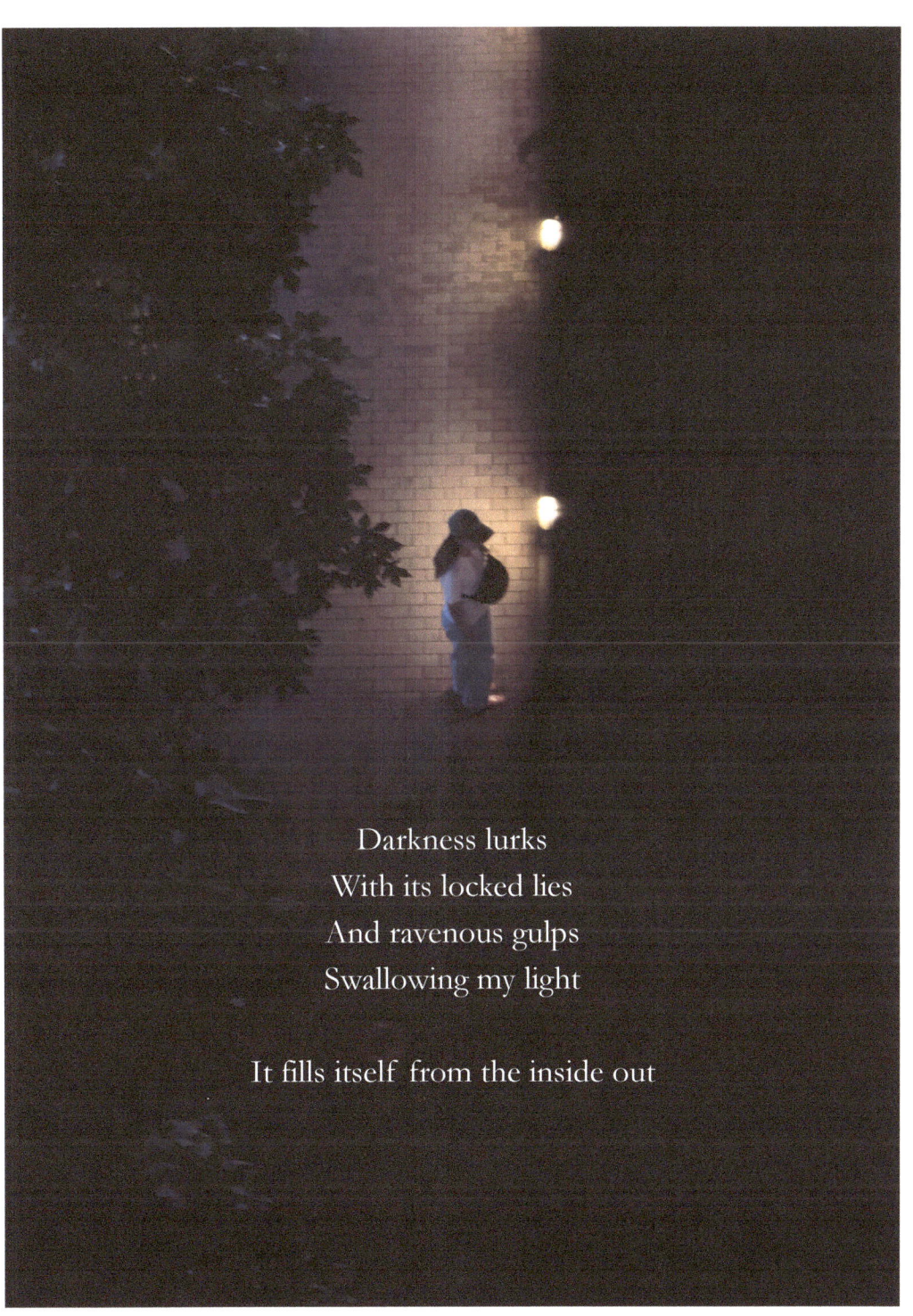

Darkness lurks
With its locked lies
And ravenous gulps
Swallowing my light

It fills itself from the inside out

losing myself

I am me no more
No more than I am you
I am nothing but a familiar heartbeat
And sore hands,
From hanging on too tight
To me.
To you.

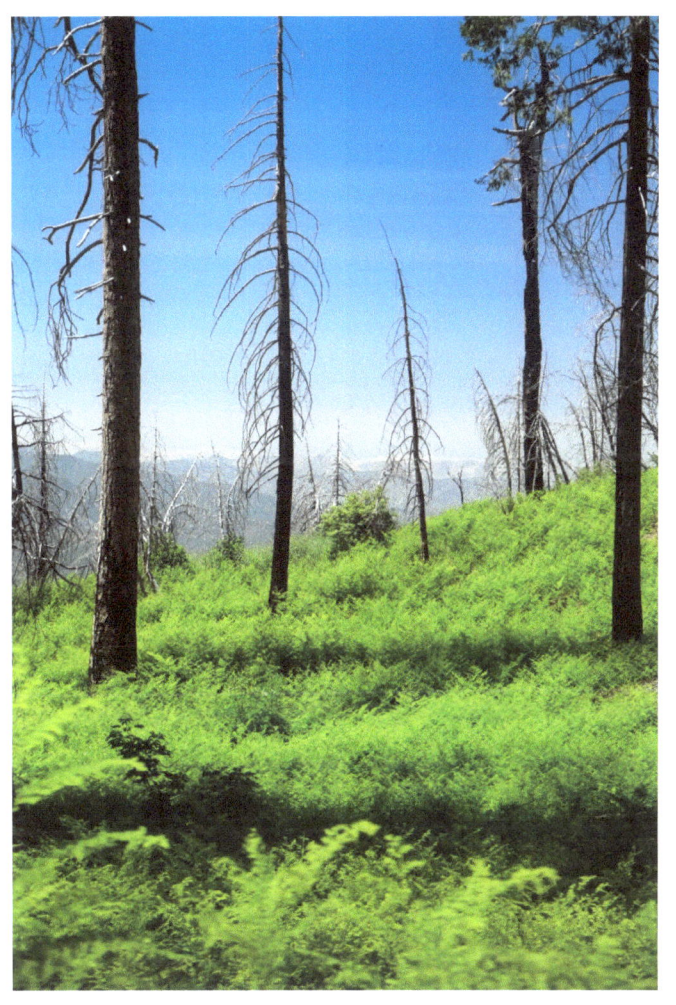

wasting away

I sway
Like a thin paper doll
Fragile edges folded
No room for a soul

no escape

Although it seems impossible
I am drowning in a drought
An arid ridden field is taking me under
Toes buried deep in its parched soil
Trying to quench my thirst
From diluted ideals
That have long since dried up

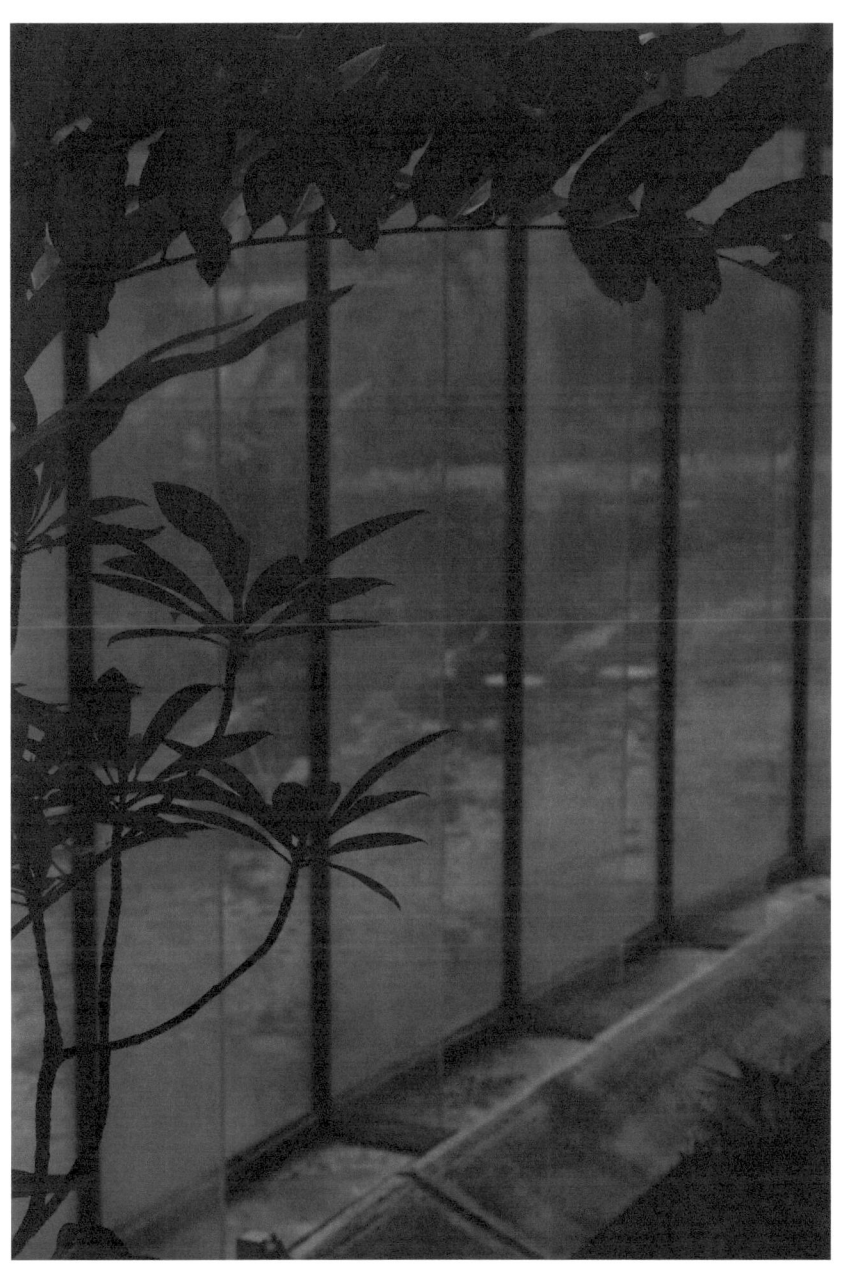

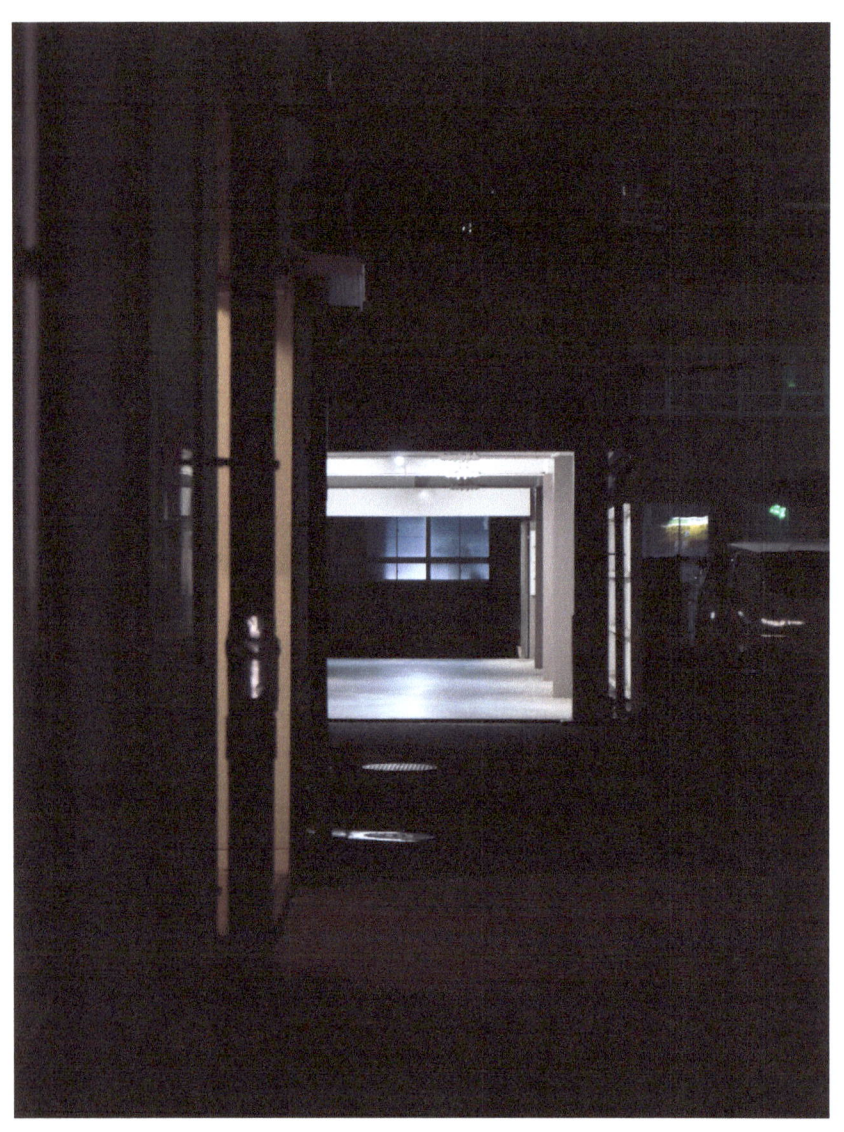

my past

Words whisper
Coming to me in the dead of night
I often wake
To find I'm in the company
of incoherent gibberish
Chaos
That I piece together
With thoughts of another time
Influenced by the people,
places and things
That were once my reality
And now
Just cloud my mind

not being enough

I wanted to be that pull
Your next addiction
That vice to keep you grounded
But I lost to your next win
And the pain that came before me
I couldn't compete with the cards you held tight
Pressed against your chest
And the fear that lingered within

trying to make you stay

I don't need another standstill
Or stop and go
I don't need another puzzle with gaping holes
Untied strings
To trip and tumble
Bending branches
Just out of reach
I've become a bag of broken bones
Created from weighted tiptoes

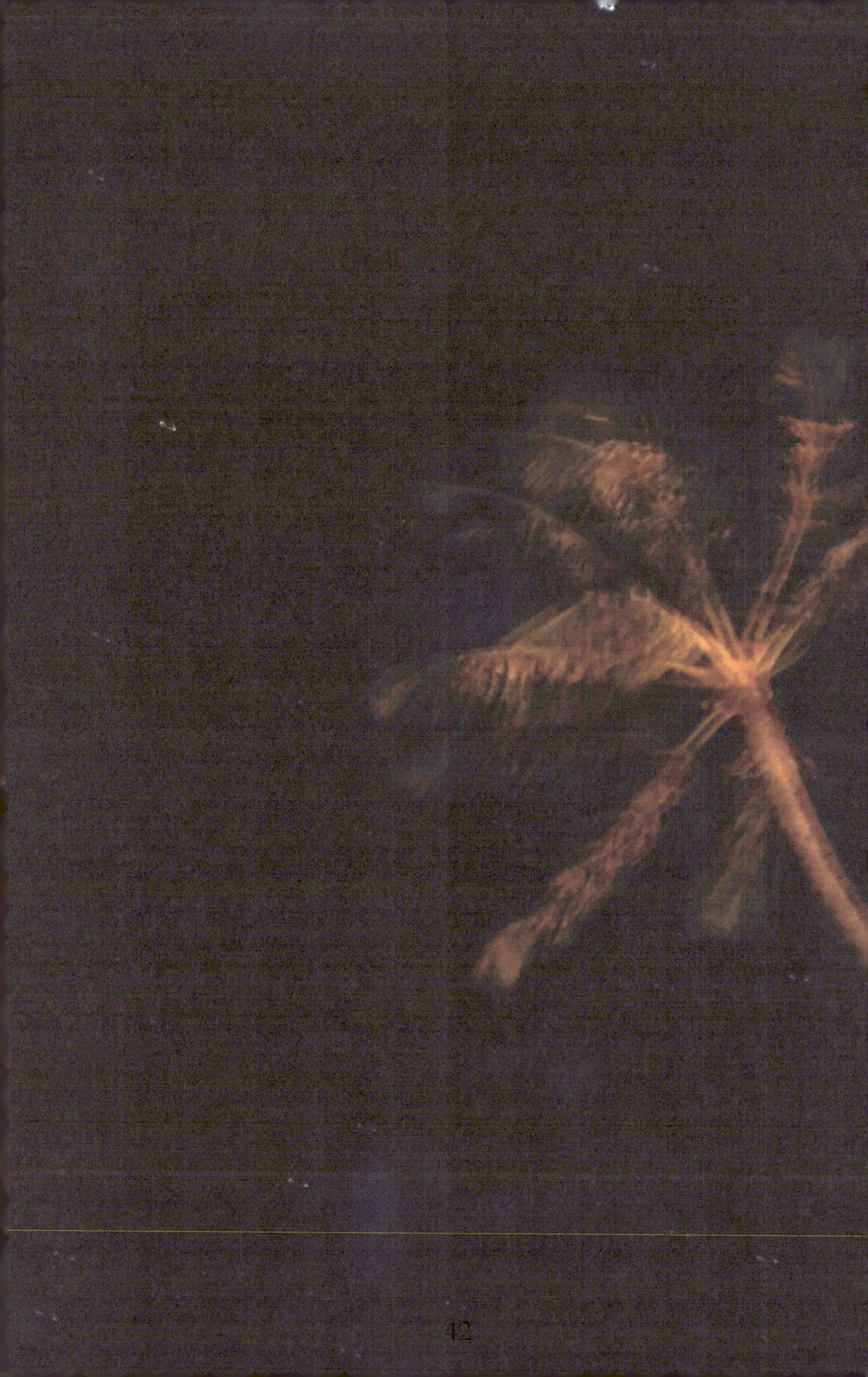

nearing the end

Seduced by midnight fog
And surrounded by the whispers of the waves
My mind afloat with sticky dew
Embraced by the light
That escaped the heavy heartache
Felt from the lonely night's sky
It stayed awake
Just for me
A speckled canvas
To give me something to wish upon
Something more
To make me hold on

losing my mind

My threads of sanity
Snag
On the sharp edges
That protrude from my broken mind

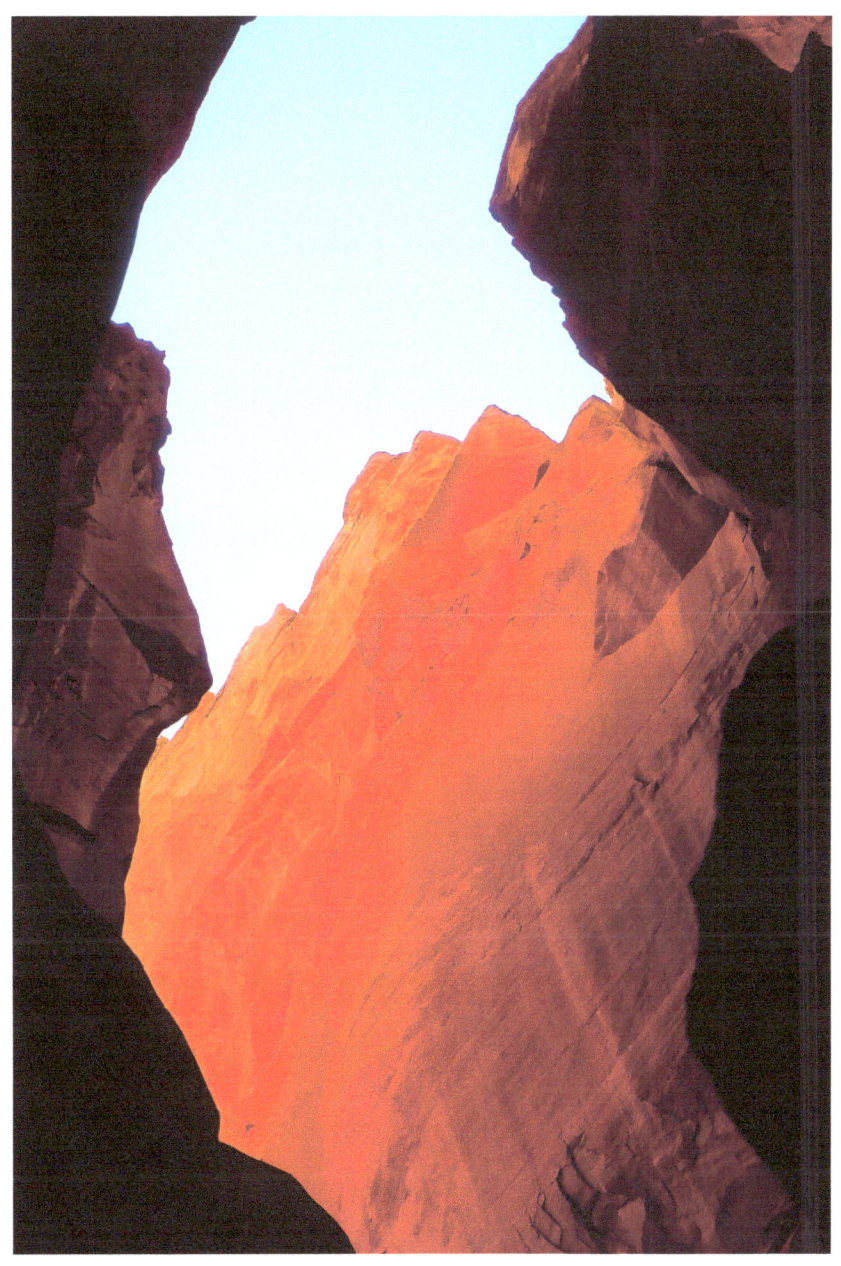

abandonment

Your inimitable attention
Filled up so much of my emptiness
But sip by sip
With eager parched lips
You have begun to take it all back
To leave me with the hollow insides
That you found me with

not seeing straight

Stumbling from too many false starts
I'm high on missed opportunities
And left unsteady by your smile
As your eyes leave me drunk on regrets

needing you too much

You were once tucked within the fluidity of my words
You were the goosebumps that lingered
The filter
That kept the outside world from seeping in

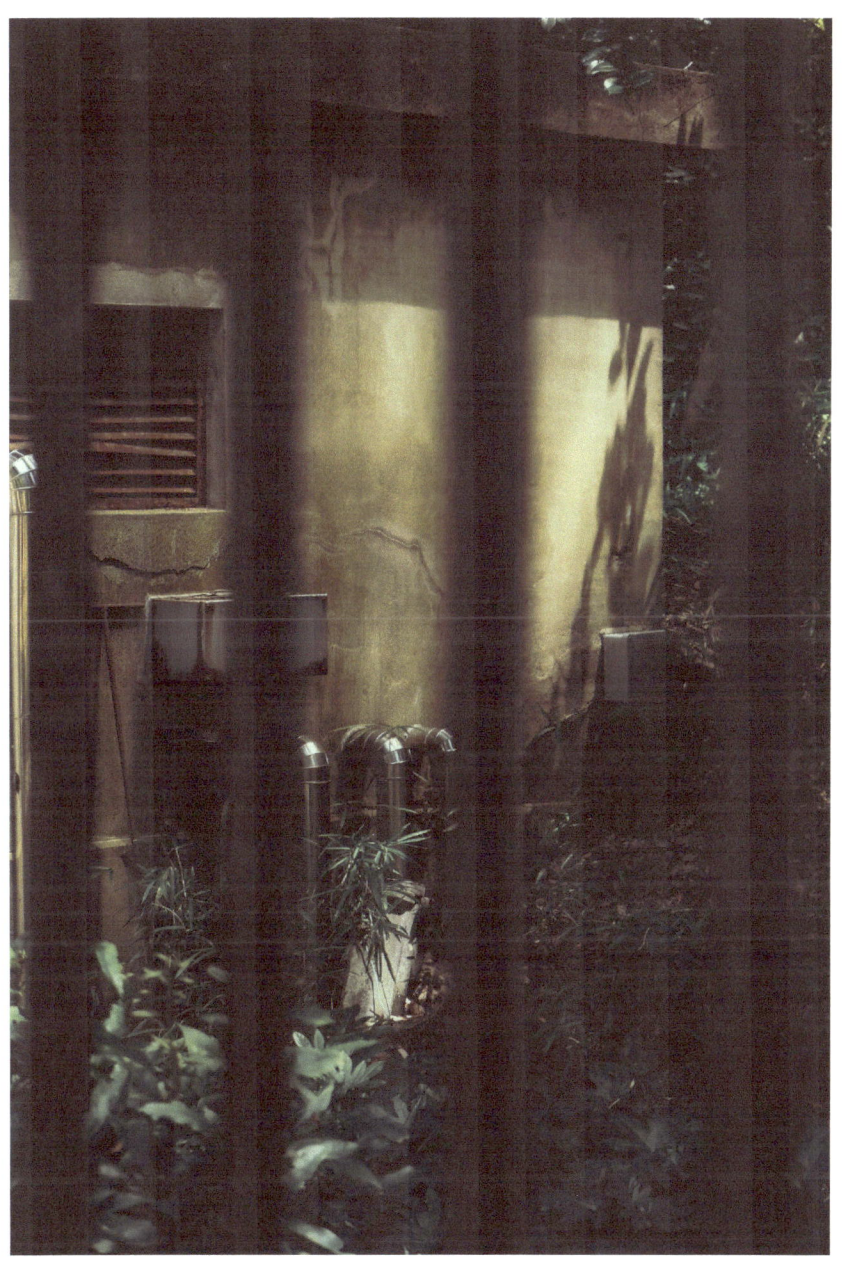

mute mornings

This cold room turns hollow
Sucked from sound

My hands
Empty
Searching to gather your warmth
From the barren side of the bed
    that was once yours

But now stares back at me
As if to say,
"I'm sorry"

charred remains of burnt bridges

Days on repeat
One folded onto the next
An accordion of time
That sings of lessons learned

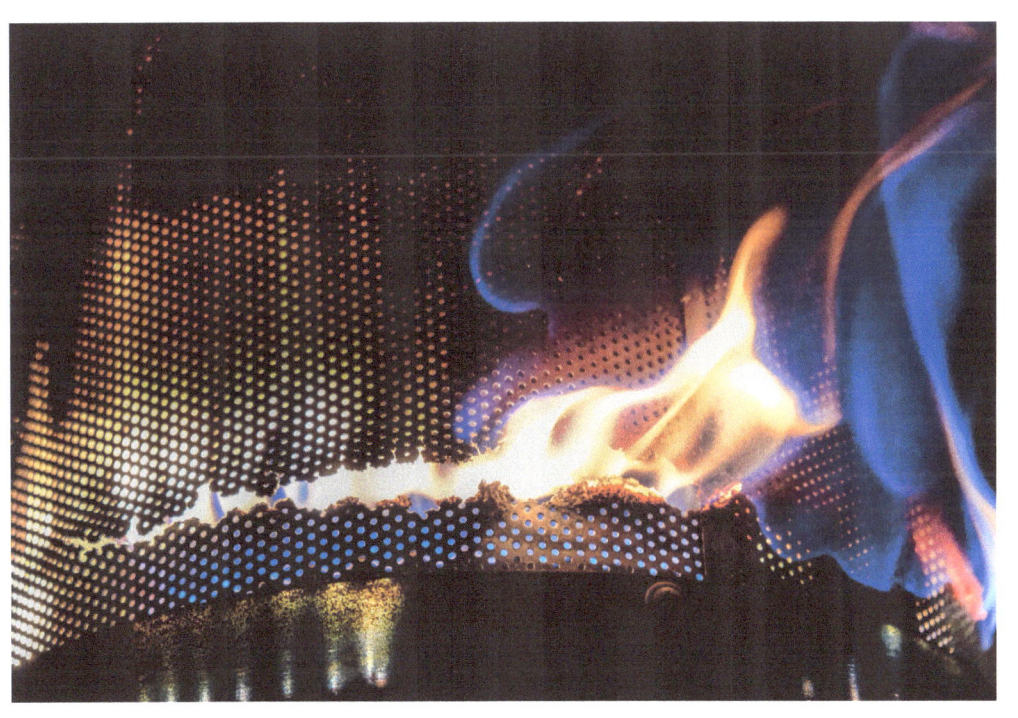

i fear it happening again

And there you stood
At the tip of my tongue
Tasting like deep blue skies
And heavy sighs

And there you stood
Falling from the tip of my pen
Wishing that we could begin again

And again

And again…

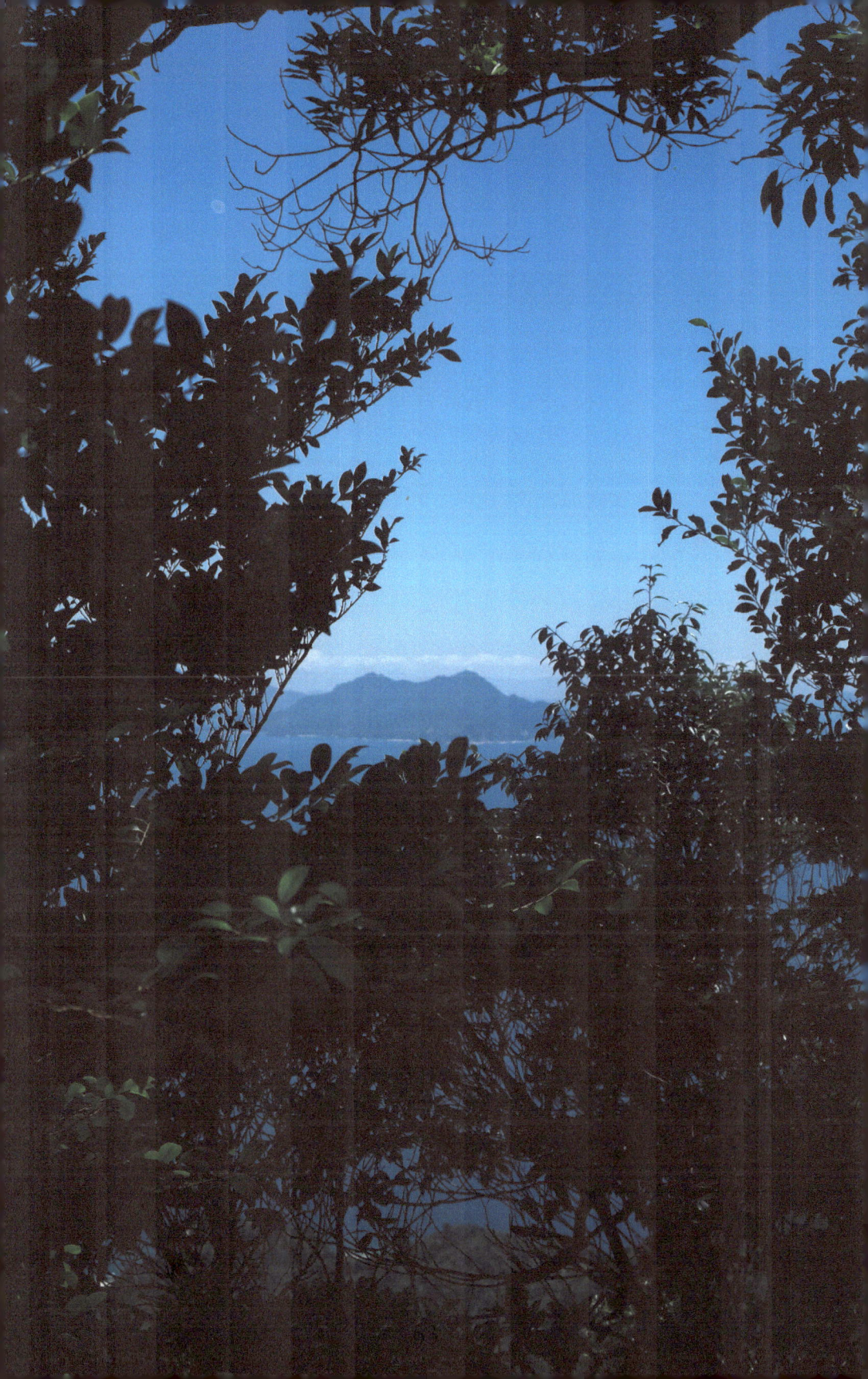

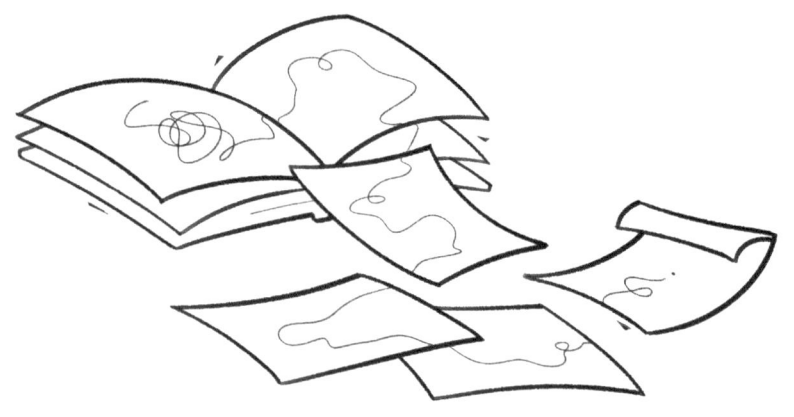

worn words

I have read our story so many times
That I can no longer tell fact from fiction
Lies from truths
We have become the cracked spine of weathered words
Peeling apart with every turn

floating away

I carry with me
Broken branches
And hollowed limbs
My withered roots
No longer holding me down
I teeter on fine fingers
Waiting for a strong wind
To topple me
Or for a wayward breeze to carry me away

losing my voice

The revolution of words
Sharp and quick
As they ricochet between us
No shield thick enough
Just this pen as my dagger

running out of time

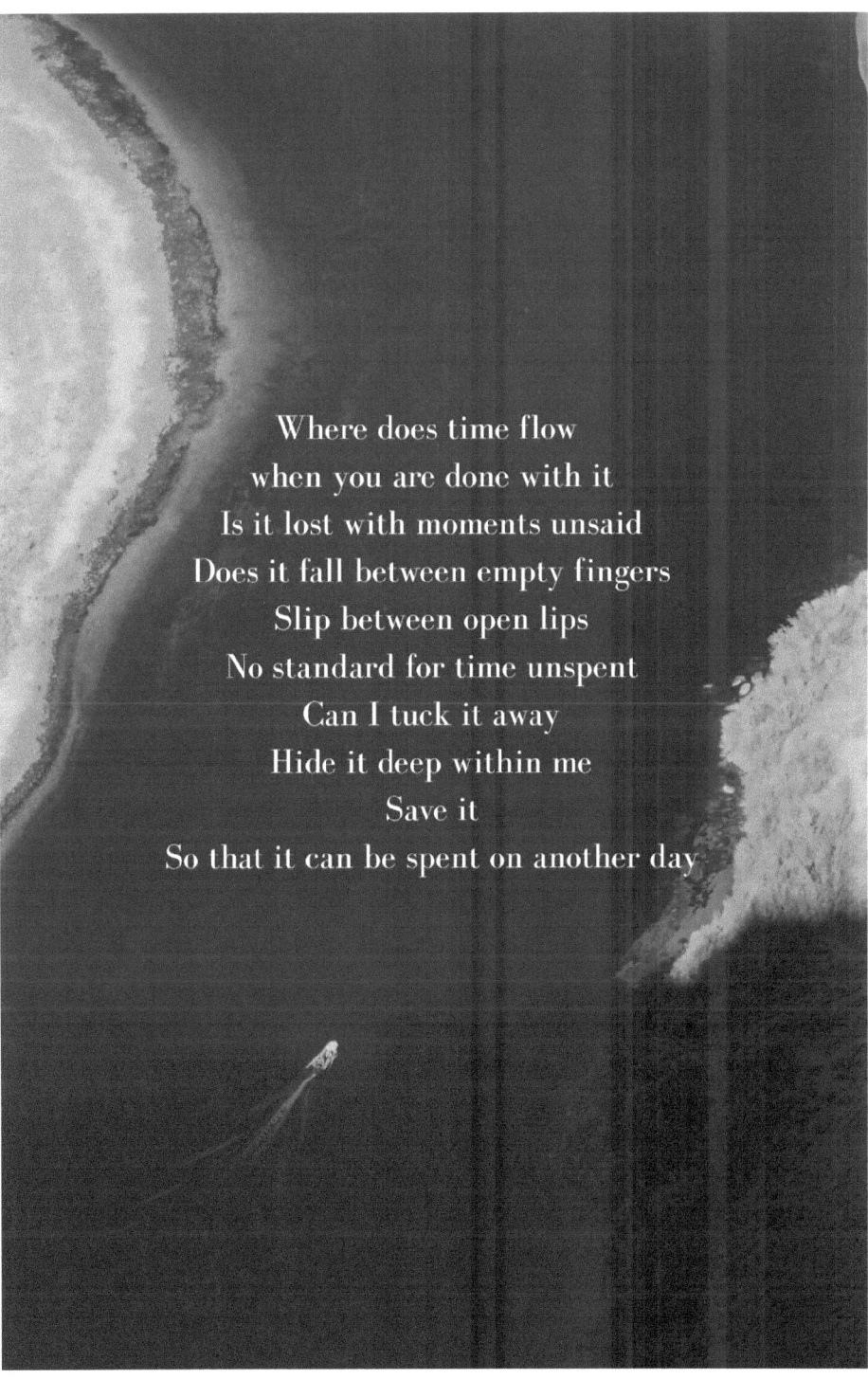

Where does time flow
when you are done with it
Is it lost with moments unsaid
Does it fall between empty fingers
Slip between open lips
No standard for time unspent
Can I tuck it away
Hide it deep within me
Save it
So that it can be spent on another day

not able to hold on

I feel the world tilting
As I climb the notches of your serrated blade
Slipping on the remains of those that came before me
You are the reason I have learned
To bend
Before I break

too much unsaid

Wishing my minds whispers
Would seep between the seams of where we lie
Plucking gently
Across our threads
To sing their confessions

feeling it all

Running for cover
Drenched in pain
From the storms that brew
And left heavy
From our last conversation
Trying to tread through rising fears
And the sorrow that I have left behind

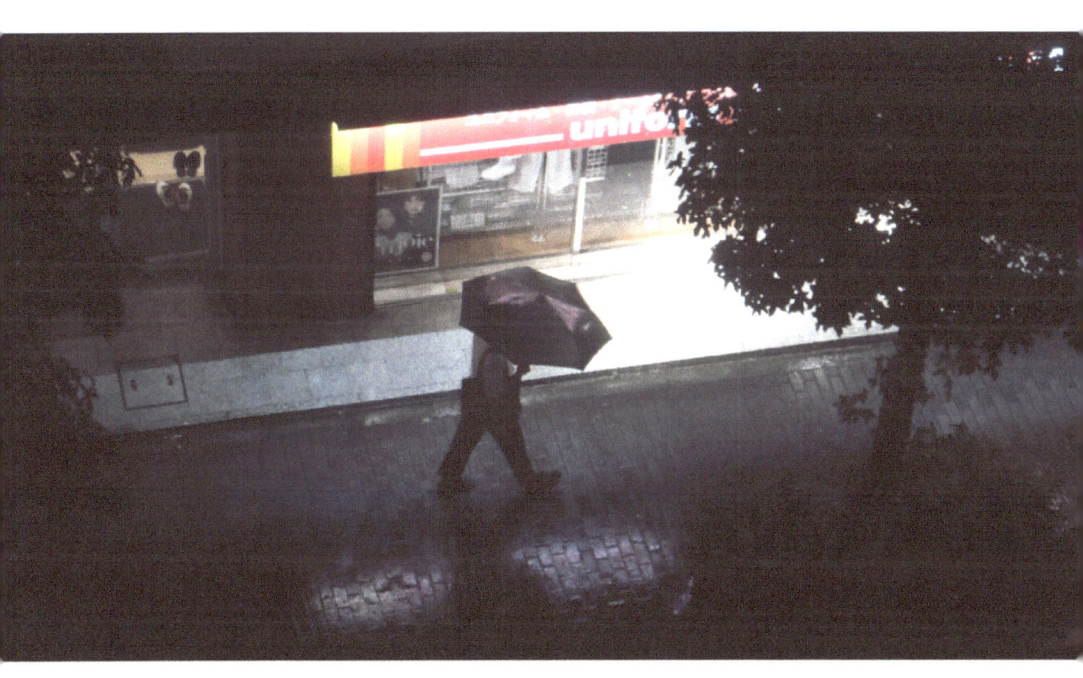

you

You're poison on my lips
A glass made of tainted crystal
I will continue to run my finger around the rim
And drink from your smile
This slow death is worth the taste you leave behind

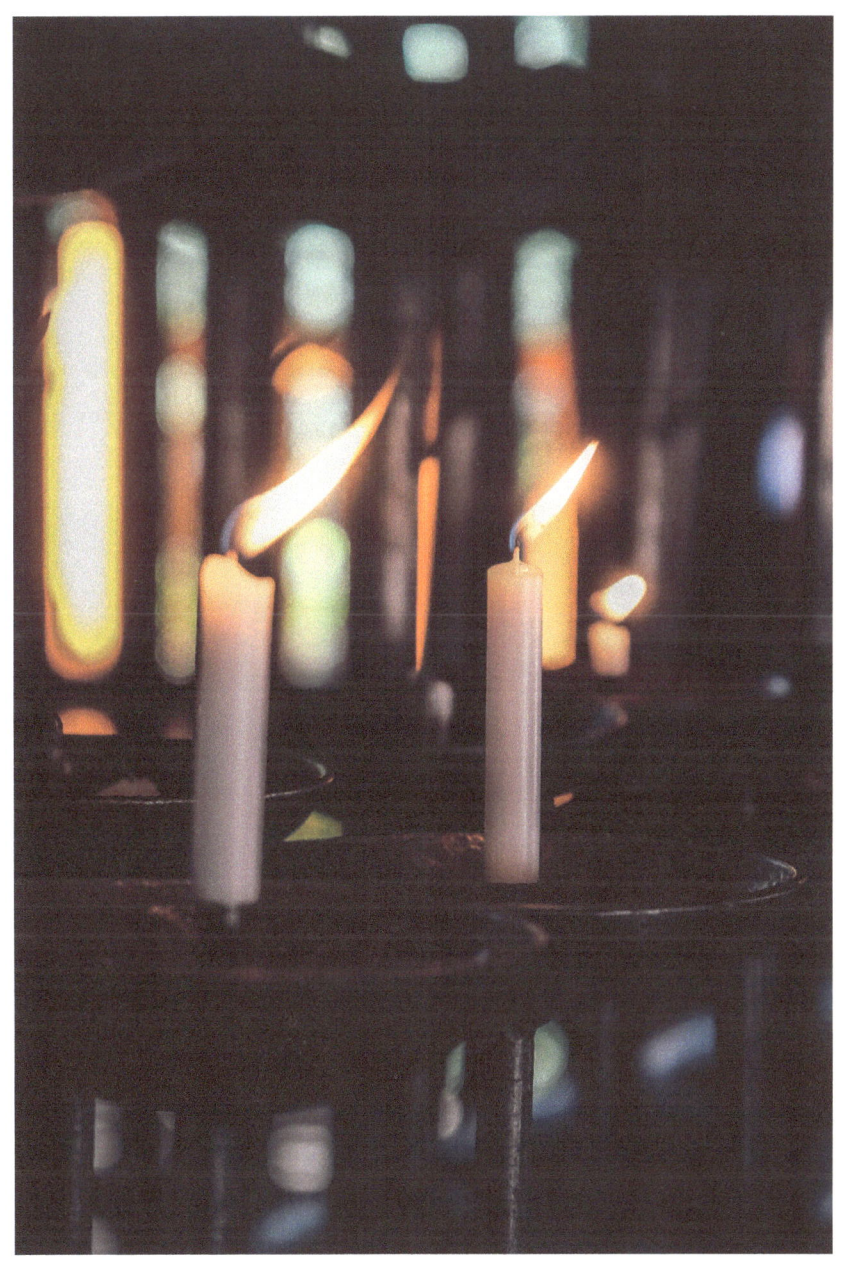

the fastest way to die

Away
Away from the sounds of summer
From the feeling of your hand
Resting upon my knee
A swipe from the stars
As they rotate overhead
Blistered skin
From needing you too much
Back bent
From holding too many memories

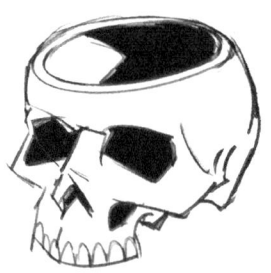

so many "what ifs"

My view of the same situation could be different than yours
My interpretation of a word misunderstood
My heart may beat at a slower pace
My mind might reel in the opposite direction
My forward could be your back
My one foot in front of the other
Might be your path to the end

disappearing

There's not enough of me left
I'm nothing more than a breath of smoke
Something you mumble in your sleep
As you lie with covers clenched
And dream of fire

not able to let it all go

Footprints follow
Shadows swallow
The past keeps pace
Through lingering memories

untruths

I see straight through you
The foggy emptiness echoes
And your lovely lies give rise to nothing more
Than your ego

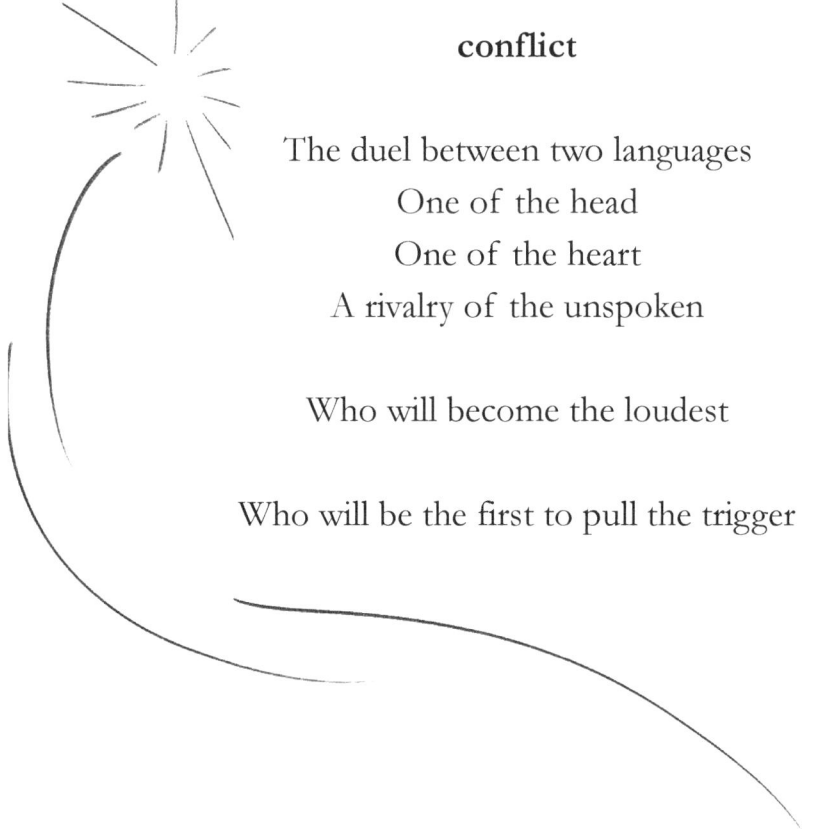

conflict

The duel between two languages
One of the head
One of the heart
A rivalry of the unspoken

Who will become the loudest

Who will be the first to pull the trigger

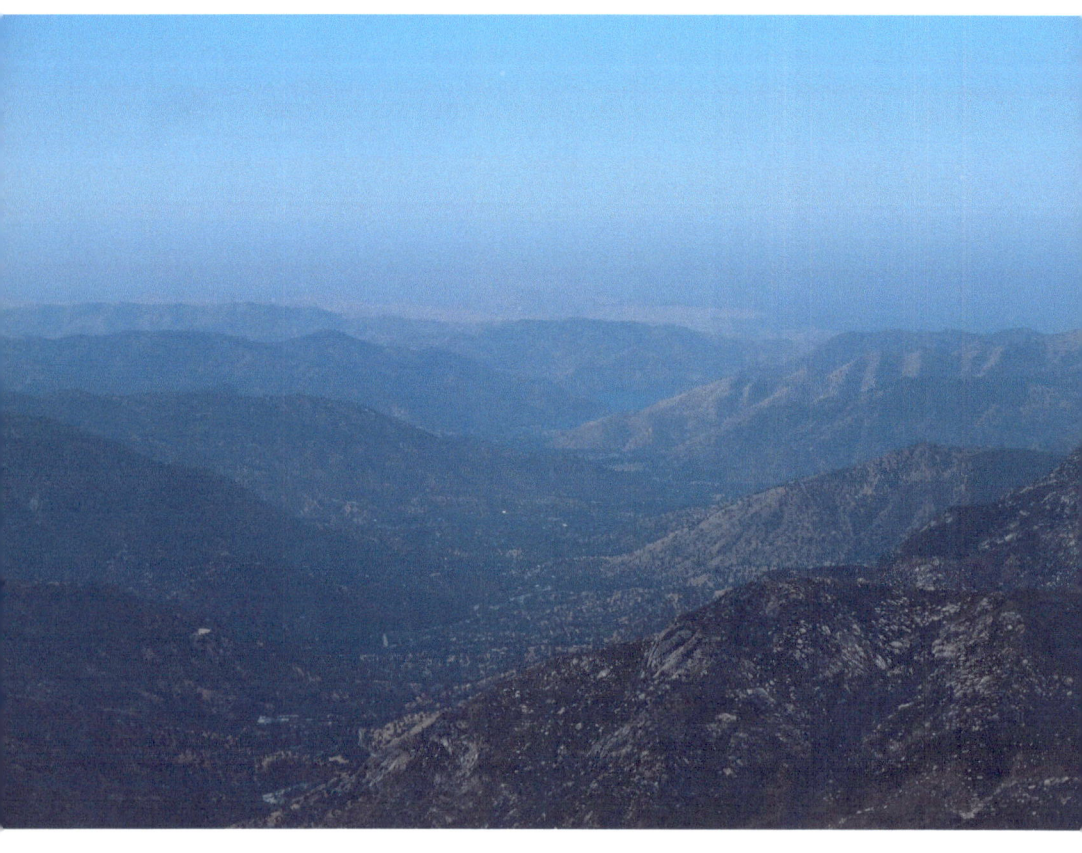

needing so much more

I want to be the rain that the clouds weep
The breath of birds
That dance in the treetops where mountains sway
I want to be the darkness
Of the shadows that fall from tall trees
I want to swim with the wild that follows the streams

remembering

I've spent years
Drifting back
To weighted mornings
That were broken by my breath pressed
Against your back

starting over

I've lost my leaves
And my ability to shade myself against the heat
Barren bones
Broken skin
Nothing left
But what dwells beneath

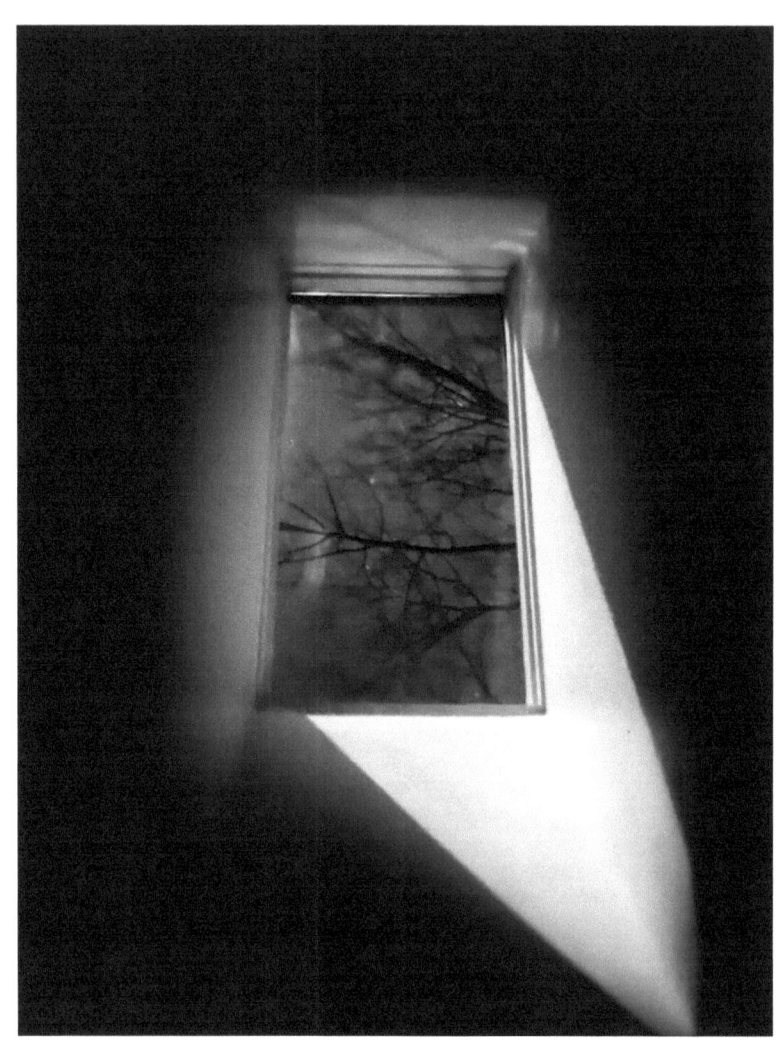

forgetting

I wear thoughts of you
Like the moon wears the reflection of the sun

relying on the night

I filled everyday running
Putting thoughts in a jar
Sealed off from reality
Not wanting to fight anymore
My mind traveling
Back to the place
Where stares first rose
And our sighs fell heavy into the night
When darkness hid our problems
When darkness was our friend

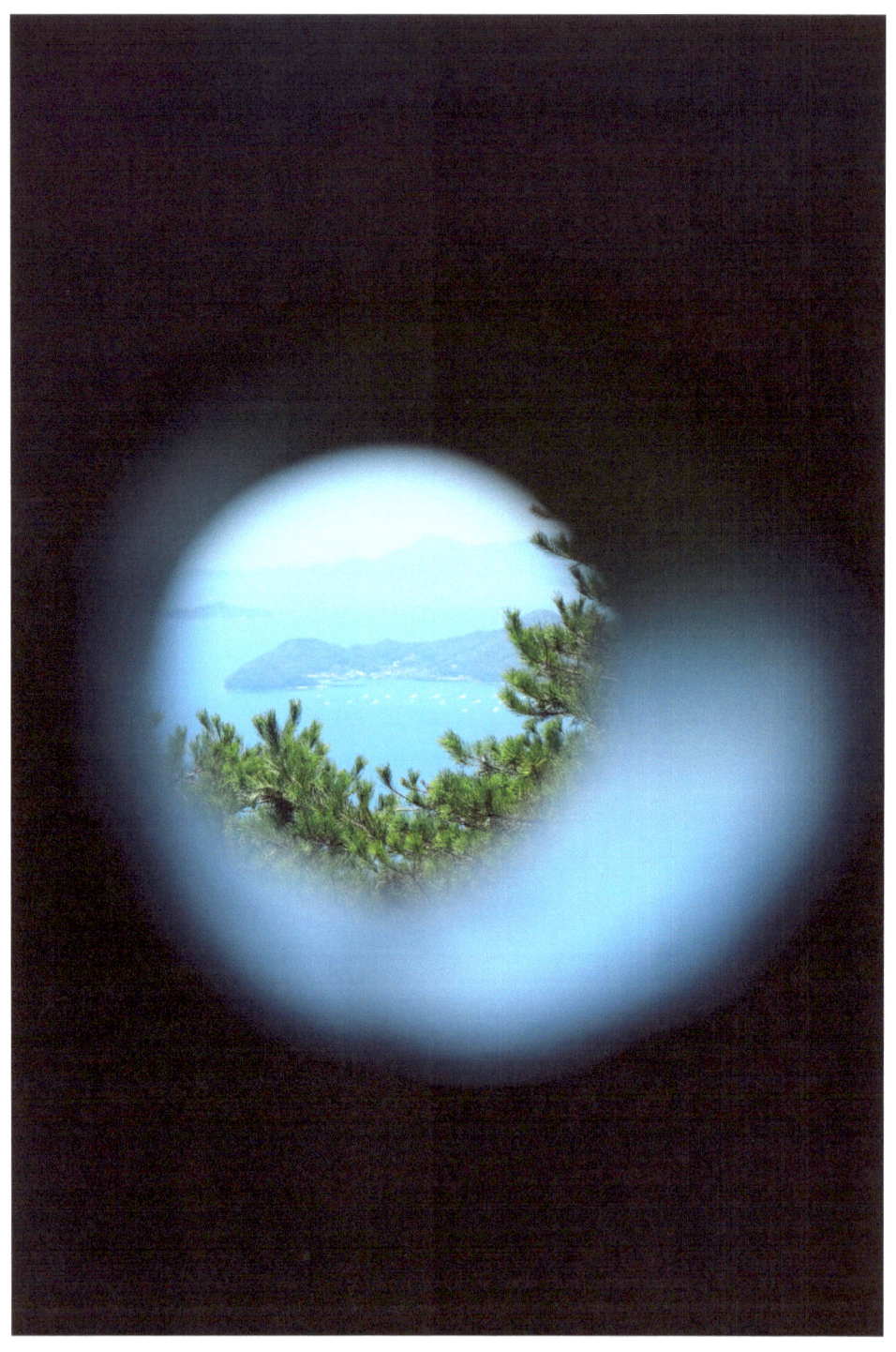

what comes next

Everything before me
Will eventually become my past

I am nothing more than the mirror in the middle
Meant to absorb everything around me

But instead
Left to reflect

hushed passion

Feelings put on hold
Numb
Stagnant hands
No longer searching for our next high

holding on

Your words linger
Passing through me like a ghost in the night
Their vibrations rattling my bones
As they settle in
To keep my mind on you
Long after I meant to forget

letting you in

You are able to tap dangerously
    into my imagination

Become concealed
    within the images in my mind

Tucked away
    where the real world no longer visits

Where I am no longer able to hide

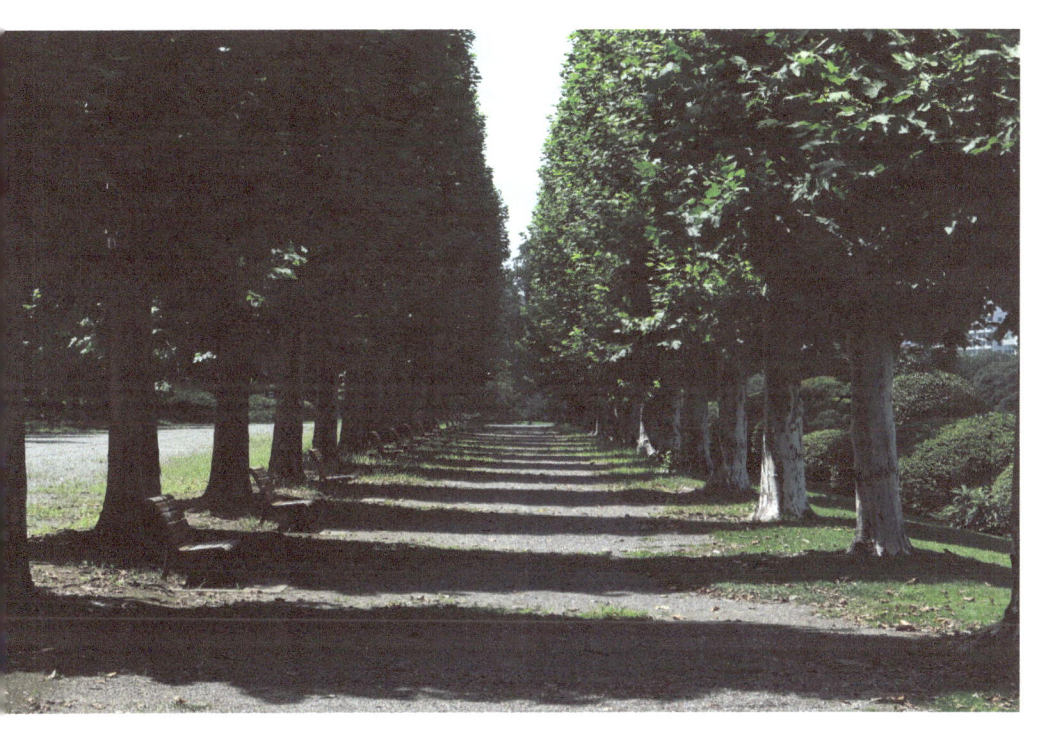

dead ends

We have become an empty space
Where people come to mourn our love
They gather tales
Scatter lies
Leave theories
That echo in our wake

"coulda, shoulda, woulda"

I don't want to die with a pocket full of "could have"
"Maybe I should have"
"Remove the fear and I would have"

our chemistry

I clutched my heart
As it morphed and moved
Pained and ached
Contorted by inexplicable alchemy
As your name filled my veins

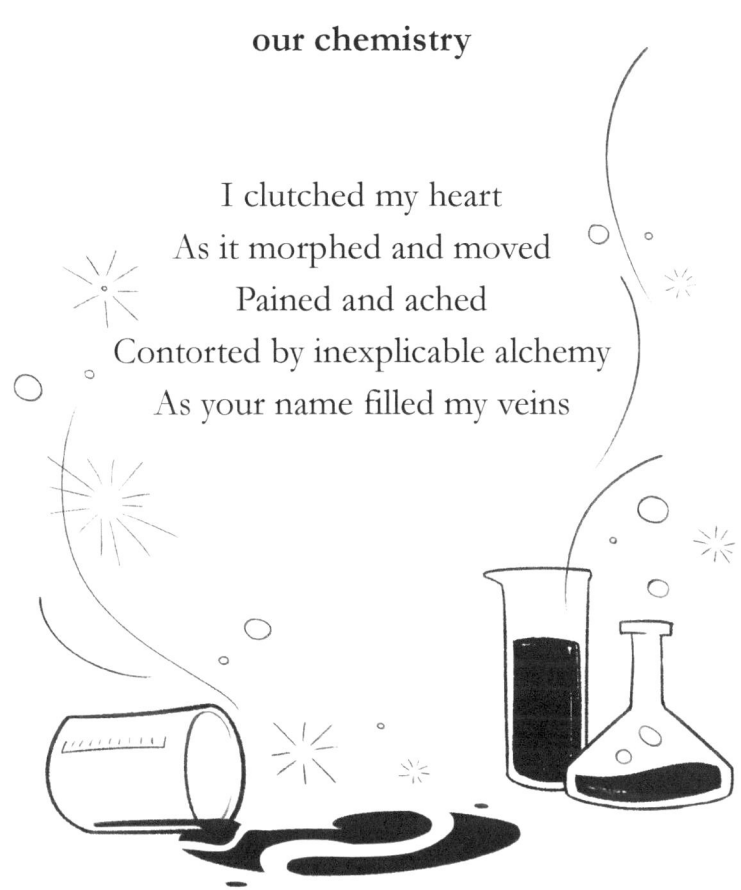

a midnight run of a racing mind

Darkness lies across my bare skin
Like heat on a humid night
Heavy with its own agenda
Almost suffocating
Taking with it any chance of sleep
Leaving behind thoughts of nothing important
But everything that thinks it should be

chasing shadows

I'm moved by the quiet
The distant applause of rustling leaves
Goosebumps form from the flutter of a bird's wings
Tears spill from watching the clouds
As they pass over and through one another
A moment of seeing them become one
And then quietly parting ways

lack of direction

I can't tell
Am I coming
Maybe I'm going
Going left
Going right
Going up
Going down
Gone
Too far gone

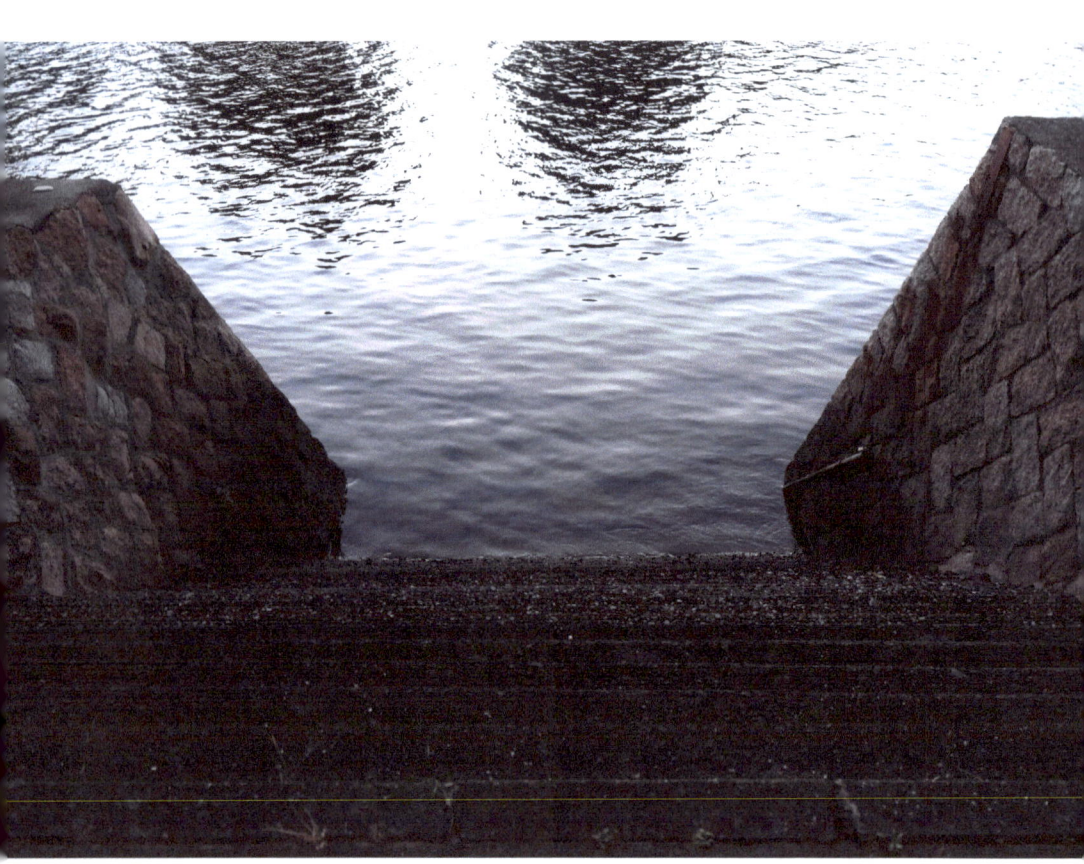

the pause

Chewed up
Spit out
My numbed mind tumbled dry
From your games and manipulations
My well of overflowing thoughts all dried up
Empty buckets raised
As I pray for rain

I'm tired of trying to be something
Someone
Who no longer exists just for me

I've tried to be all that you wish
Tried to stand still
Fight time

I need you to put out the fire
Release my mind
Transfer your desires
To someone who can give you all that you need

i fear the end

Acknowledgements and Thanks

I need to first recognize my two incredibly talented sons, Ashton and James. Your art truly shines and gives so much power to my words. Thank you for always believing in me. I am so incredibly grateful to be your mother.

A huge thank you to Christine Stephens-Krieger and Scott Krieger for believing in Grand Rapids poets and for creating a space for our voices to be heard and read. And to all of the new friends that I have made through the Grand River Poetry Collective. Each of you inspire me daily.

To my immediate family - Myron (dad), Martha (mom), Kyle, Darcie, Robyn, Tristen, Saegan, Emma, Riley, Wrenlynn, Ryann and Rowan. What a beautiful family tree this is and one that I know will always have a place for many more.

To the person who pushed me out of my comfort zone and helped me create a space where we could collaborate as artists. Dena Robles, without your encouragement to put my poetry out into the world I would have remained a silent poet who wrote just to stay sane. Now my hope is that my words will help others heal and realize that they are not alone.

To all of the poets, artists, writers, musicians and lyricists who encourage me to share my stories.

And finally, to my love, my partner, Aaron Coy. You have given me new life through your continued support. Thank you for showing me how it feels to be heard and seen. Two things that have evaded me for most of my life. Having you, Kendall, Caden and your family in the lives of myself and my boys is a true blessing.

www.ingramcontent.com/pod-product-compliance
Lightning Source LLC
Chambersburg PA
CBHW040852120626
46547CB00006B/576